Invisible War: Our Ever-changing Crisis
Volume 3 (includes 1 & 2)

Bobby Simonds

ISBN: **9798640990461**

ISBN 13: **XXXXX**

Library of Congress Control Number: **XXXXX**

LCCN Imprint Name: **Independently published**

https://www.amazon.com/bobbysimonds

Front Cover & Editing by author.

HASHTAGS:

#bobbyraysimonds

#bobbysimonds

#BOBBYRAYSIMONDS

#ATWISTINTRAVEL

#risenfromtheashes

#toxicamerica

#Challenge-thyself

#avoidinghavoc

#bobbyscreativephotography

#QUESTIONINGREALITY

#thedoctorscall

#evilmatters

#pandorasbox

#everythingchangeswithbrainsurgery

#UnfoldingMisery

#therealjerrylewis

#INVISIBLEWAR

<u>**DEDICATIONS:**</u>

I dedicate this book series, to all of you who are reading it, and have recommended it to somebody close to you! I appreciate it.

Remember, if you purchase a Kindle with me, you will have a lower-rate for returning to read/purchase your next Kindle!

<u>**About the author:**</u>

As a self-taught author, I spend much time researching many various topics. This could very well include current events, current conspiracies, and current conspiracy gossip (which I put a spin on that name).

Between using Google & Youtube; one could easily lose themselves in this long, and eventful lavish web.

I have created/published many books; which with my nonfiction, I have more than enough proof, which I can not only keep up with current events, but years later, my books seem to stay up-to-date.

Like many authors before me, I too, am exceptionally observant. I am also intrigued with the successful, mindset of being an international author, and as I continue to write, my books become more successful because of people like you, who took a chance on something new, and original to read!

I was born with Mild Cerebral Palsy, and have had brain surgery. Which, I do not allow either to slow me down, and/or get in my way. I do not compare myself to other authors, however, I do believe I have what it takes.

Booklovers connect with me from my own personal biography. Connecting with readers on more of an emotional level; I decided to include topics such as: inner healing, conspiracy, grievance, political, suicide, & finishing up with positive outcomes.

On a side note, I have assisted others to glorify their dream, by directing them with the essentials for writing, and the publishing tools, that they would need, of course.

I've soared over topics such as, social media, "fake news," UFOs, the Alien Conspiracy, "mythical" creatures, religion, politics, cloning, life-sucking tablets. Furthermore, in one book, I even predicted Donald Trumps' win, before he was even close to upsetting Hilary Clinton's supporters.

As far as my fiction books go, I must say that I am still in the process of enjoying a world to create for my readers to escape their normal bubble, to enjoy somebody else's insanity. I currently only have one true novel, and the rest being, labeled as 'novella's' or short stories. Majority of my books, both fiction & nonfiction, generally are series. Obviously, I wrote a few individuals, but I prefer the other choice.

I hope that you are brave enough to leave your review of what you had thought of with this book, and others. Whether you are a previous supporter of mine, or a new one, be respectful and leave a review where you had purchased this book. Thanks for your participation, and I look forward to reading your review, or messages to me.
In addition, I hope you (the reader) check back on Amazon.com (or whatever link you purchased my titles),

monthly, because I tend to publish a minimum of 5 books per year. Majority of the time, it's more realistically 10 books per year.

This could be anywhere in America…Coming soon, to a town near you… Introducing & enforcing Marshal Law…to you!

Invisible War: The Corona Virus Reality

Volume 1

BE READY. BE SAFE. BE HUMBLE.

Chapter 1

Wow, the world's gone crazy, no? *It's hell in a handbag!*

Well, I hope you all purchased your share of toilet paper, geese!

Living in New York has of course been up and down. Nonetheless, I had a fairly, normal life at the very beginning of March.

The day before St. Patrick's Day…everything is on lockdown…WTF? How can life turn upside down in just two weeks?

When the Corona Virus had officially spread to America, it was all laughs, until people popped up on the radar of being ill. The numbers were quite low at first, and had seemed to be mainly isolated in Washington State (Seattle). Currently, New York is being infected, thanks to the dumb folks of New York City. *And they say, city folk is more intelligent than country folk...hmmm.*

Regardless of our circumstances, life is changing drastically. Walmart and other stores were bombarded with people in search of toilet paper. Then the jokes came flooding to Facebook, and other social media sites.

I can't say much, I grabbed the last bundle of t.p., mainly because, the ass wipes went just as fast! Oh, boy, no more ass wipes? Those, work: not, t.p. Toilet paper leaves you with a crusty, smelly, hole! LOL.

Either way, then all the meat, including poultry, eggs, and deli meat became selling eagerly. Water was a huge hit, and I now wish, after purchasing the last two cases of water, that I took the offer of $300 per case, since now, Walmart restocked the water – the day before Saint Patrick's Day! Oh, well.

All weekend, I spent a good majority of my shifts standing around, doing nothing. Customers were not dining in, but using drive-thru, and stockpiling. Not much else to do, once everything is wiped down, and cleaned a hundred times over!

While standing and joking around with the staff, I had to explain what was really occurring (along with my Facebookers).

Chapter 2

What is *Mass Hysteria?*

According to *Google.com:*

*In sociology and psychology, **mass hysteria** (also known as **mass** psychogenic illness, collective **hysteria**, group **hysteria**, or collective obsessional behavior) is a phenomenon that transmits collective illusions of threats, whether real or imaginary, through a population in society, because of, rumors and fear.*

With that explained in the easiest way possible, that is what has occurred with the stockpile. That would be caused by fear, fear with not having everyday products. The other explanation from this occurring at all – at least with toilet paper, and wipes – must be in relations with *Target Marketing*. What is target marketing, you may ask? Well, if you click on an ad, or are just thinking about it (yes, you read that right), you will be bombarded with ads all day, to force you to make it all stop, you must purchase it. Radio frequencies

effecting people in the cities (mainly)
will also be affected. Yes, this is real,
not a conspiracy theory.

What comes next? I know it's
something we all say, *I don't want to
know what's coming, I could jinx
myself...* Read on, I will share my
opinions, & theories with you….

Chapter 3

The coming weeks are crucial. It's all about containment. In Oneida County, New York, there hasn't been any testing. Therefore, we cannot express the number of cases found. But what we can assume, is how many people may be walking around without the knowledge with being infected. Hence, all the business being mandatory with shutdowns. Casino's, restaurants, and gatherings are being forced down to the bare minimum with the capacity of 50 people or less, and they must be spaced out – that was, until today. All casinos are being

forced to close March 16th, 2020, no

later than 8:00 p.m. That said, I'm

officially on a paid vacation!

Oneida County is about the only

one, aside from Madison, that hasn't

had a case yet. Nevertheless, it's easy

to say, it's due to nobody being tested!

Aside from the obvious cases,

I'm not all that worried, as far as being

sick goes. Mainly because, I'm 39,

and it seems to be affecting mainly

elderly folks. Not to say, I cannot get

sick from the virus, it's just more

unlikely.

What to come, in the coming

weeks, is scary stuff. I had a vision

just two weeks ago regarding this:

1) Mandatory business shut down

2) Ration gas, food, water, and medical supplies

3) Virus Testing, willingly

4) Curfew

5) Mandatory Testing

6) Detain unwilling participants

7) Split up the infected – detainment in schools, then prison camps

8) Mass Hysteria – round 2

9) Riots

10) Marshal Law

This list is fairly accurate with my vision, it may be out of order, but I strongly believe this is what we will witness.

The conspiracy theory with this every occurring back in 2013, when people saw trains, and tractor trailers bringing in supplies such as Hummers, cargo trucks, and tanks, weren't wrong – just wrong decade. Also, during 2013, of March, *Jessie Ventura* had a show *Conspiracy Theories*, which in one of his episodes were showing empty prison camps located throughout America. The government didn't respond to Mr. Ventura's information

requests, but I can tell you for certain,

now, that they were pre-planning for

this.

The code name for the Corona

Virus is **"<u>COVID-19</u>"**. Why do you

think, 19? Was the other 18, not

effective enough? I think so.

Corona Virus disease (COVID-19) is

an infectious disease caused by a new

virus that had not been previously

identified in humans.

29

The virus causes respiratory illness (like the flu) with symptoms such as a cough, fever and in more severe cases, pneumonia. You can protect yourself by washing your hands frequently and avoiding touching your face.

HOW IT SPREADS

The new Corona Virus spreads primarily through contact with an infected person when they cough or sneeze, or through droplets of saliva or discharge from the nose.

30

I find it important to express that everyone is in a mass-scale panic. Trump is doing everything in his power to prevent the spreading of the virus, before implementing Marshal Law. But I know it's coming, it's difficult not to see it, when you have all the theories & facts racing in my mind.

Nevertheless, there will be mayhem. There will be deaths, and even casualties. We are *at war* with an infectious virus, and there isn't a cure – for the non-elite. The elite, most likely took their last stand, by creating, testing, and releasing, so they can finalize their plan with creating one last attempt for formulating, and finishing their plan; by creating a *1-world-government, a.k.a, The New World Order (N.W.O.)*. This isn't a secret, nor a conspiracy theory. This dates to the mid-1900s, and even well before that, if you dig deep enough.

Chapter 4

The signs have been in plain view since 2013. First the transportation with secret, conspiracy-like Interpol, combat-vehicles, empty prison camps, and even the strange occurrences in 'nature.' Such being, blood lakes, rivers, streams, and oceans throughout the world. Dead wild animals, that seem to be caused by a virus, that was blamed on Ebola, but obviously wasn't. It makes you wonder about the last two big scares from Virus' that were just in the past decade.

It also seems that it was always going to be ground zero, for China. Poor bastards!

China was once known for creating the Bath Salts, which caused dumbasses to use as drugs, which turned them into living zombies, eating/tearing flesh from people they encountered. Just google the man in Florida!

Clearly, zombies were a suspicion, however, they got out of the fantasy books, and moved onto something more feasible. Something that acts like the flu, but isn't.

Furthermore, making it more

assessable with the elderly, the weak,

and the young. It's what the Elite

always wanted, to wipe out a third of

the population. Just look at *The

Georgia Stones*. A man-made version

of Stonehenge, discussing the rules of

humanity.

<u>***Here's what they claim***</u>:

*1 – Maintain humanity under
500,000,000 in perpetual balance with
nature.*

2 – Guide reproduction wisely –

improving fitness and diversity.

3 – Unite humanity with a living new

language.

4 – Rule passion – faith – tradition –

and all things with tempered reason.

5 – Protect people and nations with

fair laws and just courts.

6 – Let all nations rule internally

resolving external disputes in a world

court.

7 – Avoid petty laws and useless

officials.

8 – Balance personal rights with

social duties.

9 – Prize truth – beauty – love –

seeking harmony with the infinite.

10 – Be not a cancer on the earth –

Leave room for nature.

This is to be rumored to be

constructed in the early 1990s, and was

built solely for The Illuminati,

Freemasons, and other Elite, secret

societies.

I haven't witnessed these stones in person, but I've known a few who have.

The story goes, that the person who paid for this to be constructed, made an exact replica with Stonehenge, only Secret Society style, of course. Then the man who financed it, vanished, never to be seen, or heard from ever again.

Chapter 5

Okay, I have shed light upon you, to whom haven't taken this epidemic seriously.

There have been deaths from people becoming ill with the infectious virus. Some are killed off from having a previous condition, and the virus sent their insides over the edge. However, without saying, the government is most likely only sharing a fraction of these facts. I guarantee you, that many virus-related deaths, aren't being made public, yet. I mean, why would they?

Just look at how the masses reacted with toilet paper!

Or, look at how people reacted with the radio airing with, *War of the Worlds*. You think that is a coincidence?

CONTAIN AND CONTROL. Plain and simple. We've always been the governments lab rats, and this is obviously more on a vast scale, but regardless, we're failing as a society, in a matter of days, and weeks. How pathetic!

What will become of us when they implement Marshal Law? Will it

be like that scene from *iRobot's?*
People going after the robots during
the movies version with Marshal Law?
Instead of soldiers, it's robotic
machines, that have facial features like
humans? Will we gather herds of
people to attack police or the national
guard? Just because we feel threatened
that all our rights simply diminished
with an Executive Decision?

It's obvious, that this will occur,
it's only a matter of time, and they're
using the Virus as a smoke screen to do
so. Nonetheless, at the same time, we
are out gunned, and we must bow, and

take it up our asses, as a precaution.

It's obviously a catch 22, *damned if you do, damned if you don't. Become detained or killed, survive and bow?*

Tough decisions, I suppose, only time will prove how this will all turn out.

Chapter 6

I fully understand that you may be a little frustrated that I didn't create a huge book. I simply needed to rush this book, because of the current events.

We must manage our rations, gasoline, and medical supplies. Because, another thing that could happen during these horrific instances, is that they could "reset" the button, so-to-speak.

Die Hard 4 indicates a movie-scenario in which, *what would happen if somebody just hit the reset button.*

This occurred for the Independence Day week, and it was imminent chaos! Nevertheless, this could be taken advantage of, while we are trapped inside our homes, during "self-quarantine."

I read an article about the woman who was being quarantined in her home in New York City, in which she claims that she has free will inside her home, and can only go outside onto her porch. If she were to exit her porch, and attempt to step foot onto the cities' sidewalk, they could legally shoot her. Another words, the National

Guard has "Kill-Order." Which is part of Marshal Law. If they feel threatened, shots fired, your dead. If you aren't carrying a weapon, or threatening, they (the soldier) has the option to detain you. However, the shoot-to-kill order is for those that are infected…Yep…

All I can add to this book, is be safe. Think rationally, and be well. Take care of yourself. We need to pull together, like we did for 9/11. God Bless you, and the Universe, too.

Chapter 7

Needless to say, it's been the craziest month of March, ever in recorded history. There has never, once been, a lock-down like this. Sure, there have been a few isolated cases of towns, such

as Lyme, CT. This was where the man-made disease of Lyme was created, and of course, there was an outbreak. The town was on lock-down, and at the time, it didn't become widespread. Therefore, they didn't truly get to experience, what we are today.

Beginning March 17th, 2020, many buisness were closed, by a mandatory order. It went from fully functional, to either a 25% - 75% reduction in workforce. Today, March 22, 2020, 90% of buisnesses are closed, and many people are stuck in self-isolation – before it becomes mandated with guards.

Yesterday, I was driving from Verona, New York, to Rome, New York. Generally speaking [before the virus-scare], there would be 50-100 cars on the way there, and back. Yesterday, however, it was around 10, in total. It was similar to driving thru a

ghosttown, with only the incredibly

brave motorists, driving thru!

Since my layoff, on March 17th,

2020, I have witnessed much change.

One being, Amazon's self-publishing.

This book was litterally blocked two

separate times. I'm hoping the 3rd time

is a charm, because I know the

importance of this book being released.

I shared it on my Facebook page – only

6 people to advantage with reading it

for free. However, out of those six

people, five were authors. They were

highly impressed with this book, based

on the current events. All five agreed I must do everything in my power to get the book published!

One of the last people to read it, is somewhat of a colleague – at least I would like to think so. She and I made contact a few years back with a writing group. She has written 2-3 books, which seem to be good, based on reviews & her synopsis (that I've read). I'm not a huge reader, mainly because I find myself distracted a lot of the time. It's been quite difficult for me to concentrate with writing, since bringing Jerry Lewis, home. My

Redbone Coonhound. This July 28th, he will be 2, and he is a handful. When I speak to others about him, I always say, 'he is what I call a 4-legged hurricane!'

Jerry, is our first big dog, and he thinks he is a little human!

Anyway, as you can imagine, he takes up majority of my time. Even being locked-down, with everything going on, he has been up my ass more than ever! From January 2020, until March 17th, 2020, I was working full-time as a dishwasher. Therefore, he and I didn't spend 24 hours a day with each other. Now that I am home, he not only has been up my ass, but totally abnoxious! I love him though, he is a great dog, aside from his nasty habits (tearing up furniture, watching 'daddy' clean up his messes, so he can make a new one – not a fun game).

Back to the story at hand, however, I can't emphasize enough, how many times I've seen updated press conferances concerning real news, about the Corona Virus. It's unreal, to say the least. Tonight at 8:00 p.m., is the official time for Non-Essential Lock-Down. There are new laws being implimented, like being six feet apart from another human, and only going to public places with less than 50 people as an entirety. It's strange. The roads are becoming desolate, which saves on gasoline, at least!

Because of everything occuring, majority of people forgot about Saint Patty's day, because everything was cancelled.

There has been many discussions regarding our President's "good" job. I believe President Trump is doing a great job. I strongly believe the previous two would have made this crisis much worse, than Trump. So, a special thanks to Donald Trump, for attempting to *Make America Great, Again!*

FYI: continue washing your hands, stop touching your face, and cover your mouth when coughing – that one especially!

Also, continue checking updates, because it seems to be changing every hour. Progress will be essential, if everyone does their own part.

On the other hand, be ready for looters, there seems to be a small uprise with burlaries – both home and buisnesses. Furthermore, watch for Marshal Law. There is a huge probablility that this could be your reality. If you encounter it, be sure to post "real time footage", so people are aware of the situation.

One last thing, is that I cannot emphasize enough, be aware with everything, pay attention to the media, and the President's announcements. Furthermore, watch for red-flags. There are many, this is obviously pre-planned, like 9/11. This didn't just occur overnight, they've been wanting

to have a NEW WORLD ORDER, 1-
WORLD GOVERNMENT, for nearly
a century or more. The elites, and
secret societies have finally made this
plan act out, and we're witnessing it
now. Therefore, be prepared for
anything. If you don't have/own any
guns (like myself), make certain you
aren't far from knife, for personal
protection against your predators.
Furthermore, when have you ever
witnessed the government closing
schools for nearly a whole year, over
such a thing? Not to mention, traffic
courts being closed….indefinantely?

BE READY. BE SAFE.

BE HUMBLE.

A special thanks to those whom, took the time to read this book, and all the others I created & provided for you! Your support helps me achieve my goals, with first, and the utmost important, with expanding your minds!

I special apology, to those whom may have experienced my book disappearing from Amazon's bookshelf. For some reason, or another, this book has been blocked 4 times! If I were to assume, it would be due to the reality with my theories, provided inside this book, and the next!

Invisible War: Failure to Win

STAY 6-FEET AWAY FROM ME!

(Volume 2)

<u>**A Special Thanks:**</u>

Before I begin, I would like to thank my readers for snatching up the previous book for the beginning of this series. I found it to be my number one seller for the month of March 2020; considering it was only released for the last week; considering that Amazon attempted to 'ban' my book!

Let's begin!

Chapter 1: Gloves & Face Masks

Well, it's April of 2020. What has only been around three weeks, since the outbreak of COVID-19 (a.k.a., Coronavirus) has arrived in the United States of America, life has changed drastically.

We were clearly spoiled, and now we're fighting the imprisonment of our own homes!

Before all of this came about, we all complained about getting sick, or not being able to leave – on our own behalf. Currently, every state in America has its own set of rules – most are following California & New York. However, people are no longer laughing at the virus issue. Now, everyone (including myself), cannot help ourselves (themselves) from laughing at the incompetence in America. When we must go out of our homes (risking getting sick), we must go to the bank, get a gasoline fill-up (or a partial), and stop by the store.

Lately, people have been following China's lead with wearing gloves & face masks. The issue isn't that people are attempting to take the proper precautions. It's the fact that they're not following a simple-common-sense factor.

Let's begin with the gloves. Most people wearing gloves, aren't doing anything different than if they weren't wearing them at all. There have been reports on social media, and people I know, including myself, seeing the dumbness ***grow larger than the infectious disease itself***!

People who wear these disposable gloves are touching their faces, picking their noses, and grabbing their crotches (yeah, dirty men)! Furthermore, they're touching everything from shopping carts, their vehicles (inside & out), door handles, currency, and God only knows what else – without changing from one pair to the next! You may as well just be wearing work gloves. At least you can wash them when you get home!

Okay…sigh…Facemasks. This one bugs the crap out of me, and everyone with half a brain!

Not only have I seen this numerous times (nearly every time I leave my house) in person and online; but I cannot help myself with shaking my head and laughing.

There are a few different styles of face masks to use. The obvious type is what medical professionals use, and pass out when you are entering a clinic, or the hospital when you are sick (and contagious). It's a no brainer. You take the little string parts, wrap it around you ears, the square part, goes over your mouth and your nose. Simple, isn't it? Apparently not!

My cousin and I were talking about this today, in fact. We were comparing the 'dumbing down America' factors with such a simple, no brainer thing. Like wearing a cloth mask over the proper parts of a person's face, and these people (it could be you, or somebody you know), cannot even get that right!

I've even seen people wear it on their chin. Just their bottom lip. Or just their nose, even. It's rare, thus far, I've seen a human being (at least 100 people now), wear it properly!

Another form of face mask, is the industrial kind. Like the prior mask, you cannot have facial hair – because it gaps the mask from the skin. The tightness is what keeps out an air-borne disease, bacteria, and/or fumes.

Nevertheless, the same dumbness I've mentioned about wearing the cotton mask, is no different than these dumb people wearing an industrial mask.

Here's the thing folks. Whether you have a brain (and no how to use the simple functions with it) or not, you must at least do a simple YouTube or Google Search! It takes no time at all to see the proper procedures with wearing it. Now, if I had to wear a mask, it would be the industrial version. Mainly, because it comes with (most of the time 1 set) the cartridges. They range between $10-20 for the replacements. And you technically only must change those out once a month.   As far as cleaning the mask goes. That's just as simple. The alcohol swabs/pads that we all purchase at Walmart or where ever, we use to clean our glasses or phones…well, you can use those too, for cleaning the rubber parts of the mask! You don't have to get a specialty cleaner, because, all-in-all, it's the exact same thing as I just mentioned – for a fraction of the cost!

Again, for a dude, you cannot have facial hair with either mask, or you will have a gape, which will defeat the intentions with wearing the mask. I was certified with mask wearing back in 2008-2011. It's not rocket science. A monkey can figure it out, if he/she knows where their butthole is!

Chapter 2: Social Distancing

This was difficult to adjust to. But not difficult, when you are paying any attention.

The minimum requirement for this action is literally only ***6 feet***! People waiting in line: 6 feet. People grabbing something next to somebody else: 6 feet. Entering/exiting a store, isle, or whatever: 6 feet! Not difficult. We've been all doing this for more than 2 weeks! Why is this so difficult?

I was sitting in my car just yesterday, waiting for my wife to exit Lowe's. While I was waiting, I was viewing new posts from Facebook. Then I noticed a man, yelling from across the parking lot to another man. They greeted each other gratefully, shook hands, then stood two feet apart, and talked to one another for ten minutes. Ironically, they were discussing people misusing the **_6-FOOT RULE!!!_** How can you not see, the IRONY!

Chapter 3: Lock-Down's

The lock-down's all began a week or so, after a ton of the business were forced to close. Basically, what this rule is coming down to is, well, a voluntarily quarantine in your own home. Key word: VOLUNTARILY. The issue is, that not everyone is following the pressured suggestions to stay at home, and stay inside. I can't, myself, and I used to be home all the time. It's as though, since they are pressuring us to stay home, we cannot.

Simply put, if you are trying to climb a very tall ladder, and the person attempting to encourage your

braveness says, "don't look down."

What do you suppose will occur? WE

ALL LOOK DOWN. For some

strange reason, that is total instinct.

And, quite honestly, I believe that is

what is occurring with this situation.

We cannot stay home, because

we were told to. And as children (yes

adults too), we do the opposite! Then,

when American's don't get their way,

what do you suppose the 2nd thing

occurs? We act out!

Anyway, Pennsylvania went into

total lock-down, shutting down all

businesses; including the non-essentials or whatever, workforce. I believe New York will be next; because we have the highest death count; including infections. The issue is, that the numbers are lower than what the reality is, because they're not testing everyone – as they should be. As President Trump insisted a suggestion for (which I thought of days prior), is an ***at-home-test-kit!*** All they need to do is charge a dollar for the test, and it will be more precious than toilet paper!

The issue is, once everyone does get tested, that doesn't mean that it's the only time they will have to get tested.

Let's say, that I'm healthy. I get tested, and I have a great result, with not being positive. Now, two weeks later, I get the symptoms. You know the basics: trouble breathing, dry cough, high fever (no pins & needles). Then, I must get retested, and now, I test positive for having COVID-19. Then, you will have the media throw a spin on the story, by saying something about the first test, being a false-positive (like pregnancy tests for women). Then all hell breaks loose, and people will claim that the tests are legit. So much drama! But it's true. If you test negative, you can still test positive down the road. Rich or poor, powerful, or not, this is a simple fact.

Therefore, taking precautions could better your odds with not getting sick in the first place. Think of those idiots in cold states – like New York, wearing nothing but a t-shirt, shorts, and sandals in the middle of a blizzard (which I've seen plenty of times); and

then what do you suppose happens?
They get sick!

If people took the **6-FOOT
DISTANCING RULE MORE
SERIOUSLY, THE ODDS WILL
DECREASE!**

And, because not a lot of people
are "practicing" the social distancing,
people are continuing with becoming
sick, some are dying, and the rest of us,
who are following the social distancing
rules, will suffer the consequences with
losing any type of freedom during
these horrific times.

Then there will be a full **lock-down** set in place. With the obvious: detainment, unnecessary killings from Police or the National Guard (from fear of becoming sick, because you cannot follow a simple request).

I wrote in my previous book about the high possibility with Marshal Law. This is what I was gearing toward, as a point. If you cannot follow a request, nor enforced rules – once they must go that route – what do you suppose their next step will have to be? **A shoot-to-kill order?**

Marshall Law? Detainment?

Choose one, any are possible, and

scary as hell!

Chapter 4: Unemployment <u>CHAOS</u>

Because our government forced 80% or so of the countries businesses to close, that forced millions of people (including myself now) to file for Unemployment Insurance Benefits (basically means Unemployment Paychecks). The greatest thing Trump did, was add an extra incentive pay for 18 checks/weeks to your unemployment. And it went from 2-thirds of your paycheck, up to 80%. Therefore, majority of us minimum wagers, will make more on our paychecks being unemployed, than if we were working our butts off with 40-hour work weeks (or greater). Obviously, that sucks for those of who are stuck working, and are being forced with new rules daily. Nevertheless, I believe the reason wasn't to keep people from not being broke – it's to put back into the economy, so the country doesn't completely tank – economically.

It's genius. **KUDDO'S TO <u>#TRUMP!</u>**

There are 4 main issues with filing for unemployment. You must do it online. I would suggest having somebody assist you with the form,

like I did – they make confusing A.F.!

Alright, you finished your

application – after the webpage didn't

load properly for an hour! Congrats.

That part's over, put it behind you…

Now, it's time to call that

number to confirm with a "human-

being" that you didn't scrutinize

yourself, in-order, to receive

unemployment benefits – and to make

sure everything was completed as

necessary.

You pick up your phone,

knowing that you will be put on hold

for hours, because let's face it, 4 million people filed this week, and it's only Wednesday!

First attempt: busy signal. Hang up. Dial again. Second attempt: "We are experiencing a high number of calls, please try again later." Click. You look at your phone, and say, "seriously?" You sigh, take a deep breath, then redial the number. Your third attempt: You get a robotic voice, asking for you to press 1 for English, 2 for Spanish. *I press 1. Next, "using your keypad, please enter your valid social security number. Okay xxx-xx-

xxxx. Got it. "Please enter your 4-degit pin code. Okay, XXXX. "Please stay on the line, because of the high volume of calls, our operators may take longer to get back to you…" You feel as though you are getting somewhere. *Lame music begins to play, then…wait for it, wait for it…CLICK! You look at your phone, and you were disconnected.

Aggravating, right? What I did, is cuss for five minutes after the 98 times I went thru this on the first day. Then I went online, looking for feedback about this issue, sure enough, the first 5 threads on Google.com –

Between 4,000 and 5,000 calls, and

you will hear from a human being –

which only takes 5 minutes of what

you are expressing in your mind as

aggravating assault charges (then you

pause, and are thankful it's not in

person!).

I was so pissed I sent the

Governor a lengthy complaint,

explaining exactly what I expressed to

you, with the frustrations. I also

suggested (which I hope they do this),

to get rid of the phone calls

completely. Once the online forms are

complete, it should show the number

of which you are in-line to wait, before

speaking to somebody via video. This

would save so much time, and

aggravation!

Chapter 5: Economic Survival

Since Trump's **Stimulus Package** was officially signed – last week; everyone saw light at the beginning of a dark, and scary tunnel. Without work, there's no money – especially since it's taking forever to finalize your online paperwork for Unemployment. Therefore, there are a ton of people (nearly 90% in my large trailer park alone), which both the husband & wife aren't making a penny, from the loss of their jobs – and Unemployment being so foolishly run.

That said, when the Stimulus package was approved, and everyone under $75k a year (based on income from 2018-2019 tax filings), were told that they are getting $1200 for each adult, plus $500 per child (under the age of 17), people were psyched! Who wouldn't be? Even though my wife and I don't have kids (only dogs, who act-out as bad teenager boys), we still will receive $2,400! Quite impressive. I did the math with unemployment, too. We will be making double with her income (and incentive pay, for working), plus my unemployment!

Savings, home improvements, a riding

lawn more, the Vet for the pup, and

savings – woot, woot! Holla!

How can one say no, with being

out of work? Sure, the beginning

process is a pain in the keester; but it

seems like a good pay-off, and/or bribe

to stay at home – at least 5-6 days out

the week – before it's truly forced

upon us!

Chapter 6: The infected must stay home

What's been pissing us a ton of people, is those whom are infected, and decide not to self-quarantine. This is now a law, folks – for all states; as it should be. It's better to be stuck at home, rather than a hospital that you cannot be helped, or jail – is it not?

Last week, in Wampsville, New York (Upstate New York, nowhere near New York City, by the way); a couple were tested positive for COVID-19. It wasn't a severe case, but still highly contagious, to say the least. These bungholes decided to leave their house, go into stores, like Walmart, where my wife works, parks, and other places, while being infected. This is how others are getting sick. It's contamination! This is the reason why it's becoming hazardous being an American. People aren't taking this seriously, and others will die.

Just after New York State went into "Lock-Down," a large birthday party in Rome, New York (again, not far from where I live), took place. According to online sources, it was to celebrate a 77-year-old woman's birthday. Nobody took it seriously, of

course (the social distancing rule/law),

and two people became infected.

Ironically, it wasn't the elderly woman,

as one would assume. It was a 34-

man, and his 15-year-old daughter.

Fortunately, out of a 30-person group,

it was only two people.

The arrival of the medical Naval

ship in New York City, had a large

heard of dummies arrive to show

"respect" to the Naval Medical crew.

Everyone didn't practice the 6-foot

distancing; because they all wore

gloves and masks. This is the type of

foolishness that is occurring around the country – not just New York City/New York state.

We all blamed China for not just creating the virus, but the spread, too. I knew right off, that it was man-made, and was released on purpose – as China had just admitted the end of March 2020. It's sad that governments create, then use their virus' for their civilians as live-lab-rats.

Nevertheless, America has shown racism and hate toward not just China as a country, but Chinese-American's, too. Martin Luther King,

Jr., would be so angry with how long his million-man march, didn't make much of a difference – except on paper. Regardless, just remember, not everyone in America is racist – I for one am not. I know I'm a mut, so how could I be racist. It would be like being racist against myself! Ha-ha.

We need to shine light upon humanity, and see everyone as one race – not individual races. We are all humans. We all bleed red, we all have the same organs. We need to be looking out for one another, even if it's from **<u>6 FEET AWAY!</u>**

I realize this book is just as short, as the previous. I also, realize, how difficult it is to detach oneself from the news updates, social media posts, and games we're suddenly addicted to these last few weeks.

I write a book until my gut suggests to me, that I know when done!

Thanks for continuing my dream by reading this book. Please take a moment to leave a review, and, look thru my incredibly large catalog of books that you may find interest with reading, during these harsh-times. Be safe, be courteous, and stay **6-FEET AWAY FROM ME, AND EVERYONE ELSE….! LOL**

On a side note, I must inform you, that not only did I experience "banning" issues/experiences with publishing Volume 1, but I did, also, with Volume 2. In fact, they will not allow me to publish a paperback with them (Amazon). Why they allowed the Kindle to be published, but not the paperback (same content), is beyond

my understanding. Even when I

questioned them (in an email), they

"stood by their decision." I don't

know. Here goes for the last volume!

Fingers crossed!

Invisible War: The Everchanging Crisis
(VOLUME 3, INCLUDES ALL 3)

Chapter 1

Here I go again, stirring shit up, right? LOL. I know, but it cannot be helped. It's been a long, boring, and everchanging life. We've all experienced similar circumstances.

Workers (Essentials), all had the constant new policies in play. And, the Management team with any company were just as confused as the normal associate. One minute it's this way, the next hour, completely different! This was the way for the first month.

With everyone out of work, the millions who had to rush to the

Unemployment Website, all had the same unjust experience. Cursing at the phone, the internet, and shaking their heads with complete wonder, with:

"How did we make it this far, as a human race!"

The incompetence was, and still is, at an all-time high. People clearly have lost their minds, along with any remaining common-sense, they once had…just a little over a month ago!

The week of March 16th was basically the week that had marked the "suspension" order. Where America, and the rest of the world ultimately went into shock-and-awe, and was

forced to stay-at-home, to self-

quarantine. Nearly 1 ½ moths later,

we're stuck in the same boat, receiving

stimulus package-checks,

unemployment (majority) deposits, and

spending it all on past-do bills, new

televisions, entertainment consoles,

cameras, and God only knows what

else.

Grocery stores are pretty much

back to a fully-stocked store. People

are forced to wear masks – some

gloves.

Then the *Power of Stupid*
occurs: 1 hand holding the mask, when
it doesn't cover the nose…or both –
your nose & your mouth! People seem
to be complaining about how the
Unemployed are making too much
money – the added $600 per week.
Meanwhile, Trump is pushing (or has
pushed) a *bill* to add $2,000 per month
to already employed workers, for up to
six months.

Meanwhile, nearly every state in
America, has, or will be, filing for
bankruptcy. New York has announced
that they don't have enough money to

pay for the millions of unemployed

workers, and urges Capitol Hill to send

more money. In the meantime, Trump

and Governors urges one another to re-

open the country, to send people back

to work.

Back at the end of March, the

government claimed that they won't

re-open America until they come up

with enough tests to have everyone

tested. Then, they claimed before

sending people back to work, they

wouldn't do so, until they came up

with a vaccine. Currently, it seems

that Money is the only true motivation.

Because, all-in-all, the death toll is way

under than what they claimed it would

be; and, they don't believe we will see

another "wave" until September of

2020 – which would last until March

of 2021.

Chapter 2

The inflicting fear being forced into American's, is unreal. Fake news and the *misinformation* stage is an uproar, and at an all time high. There are fear-loathing folks that believe pretty much anything, because of the amount of fear, stress, and lack, thereof, of being outside in the world, is astonishing.

Recently, face-masks became mandatory while entering any type of establishment, and they encourage (should force) the 6-foot, social distancing thing.

There are many things that are changing. It also looks as though, that I have been proven correct, with my notions that we won't be going back to "normal." Believe me, I wish I wasn't right about that, but I am, so, *I told you so!*

Our Constitutional Rights are being stripped by the day, and that wasn't going to surprise me. Look below (at the image), and see for yourself, that it was part of the plan, all along.

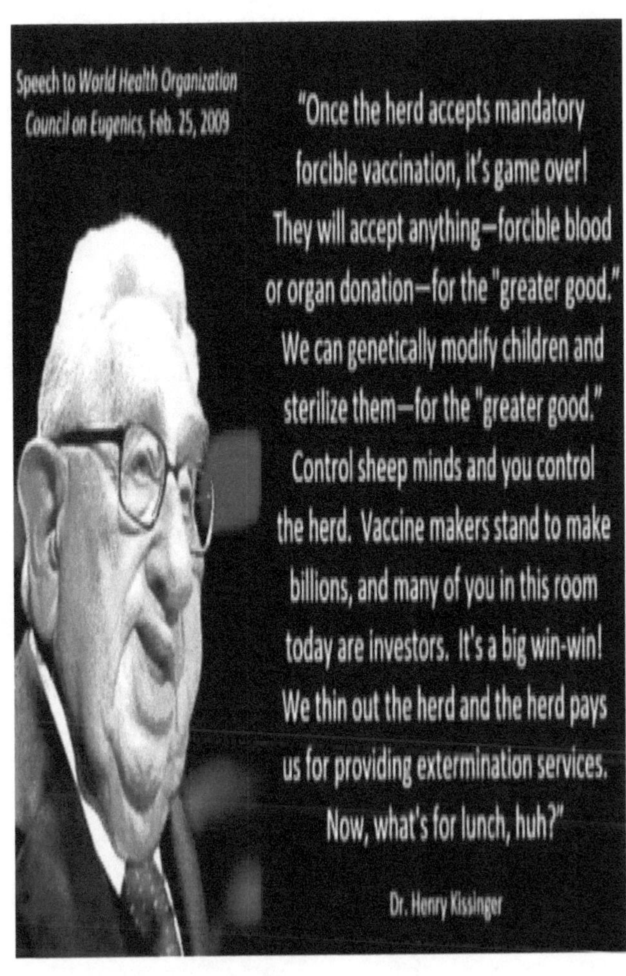

It's clear to me, after seeing this

online, that this proves, that *They – the*

Elite – have been planning this all

121

along. Even our previous President,

Obama, had a speech, urging to finance

a plan to counter-act an *Impending*

Virus.

Furthermore, a science lab in

China, had 'created' this virus. The

nickname is COVID-19, *WHAT*

HAPPENED WITH THE OTHER 18?

Chapter 3

With millions of families being home, including their once, schooled, children, many are using tablets, cellphones, and computers. The lag is unreal with online video games, and kids that went to school, just six weeks ago, are become resilient with their tablets. Check the following image I had found, that fits the criteria for what we're experiencing!

Aldous Huxley was an English Professor & Philosopher from 1894-1963; which he said:

"There will be in the next generation or so, a pharmacological method of making people love their servitude, and producing dictatorship without tears, so-to-speak. Producing a kind of painless concentration camp for entire societies, so that people will in fact have their liberties taken away from them, but will rather enjoy it, because they will be distracted from any desire to rebel by propaganda, or brainwashing, or brainwashing

This is exactly what is occurring

as of today, and since mid-March of

2020.

On May 21, 1992, Henry

Kissinger spoke in an address to the

Bilderberg meeting at Evian, France.

This has to do with "the plan." Here's

what he stated:

"Today, Americans would be

outraged if U.N. troops entered Los

Angeles to restore order; tomorrow

they will be grateful! This is especially true if they were told there was an outside threat from beyond whether real or promulgated, that threatened our very existence (Covid-19?). It is then that all peoples of the world will pledge with world leaders to deliver them from this evil. The one thing every man fears is the <u>unknown</u>. When presented with this scenario, individual rights will be willingly relinquished (surrendered) for the guarantee of their well-being granted to them by their world government."

Wow, doesn't that hit home a bit? This is exactly what is occurring, today…not tomorrow, today. And we are allowing this to occur, due to the Coronavirus.

Bill Gates recently suggested that when the Coronavirus Vaccine is official, we need to come up with a tracking, whether it'd be a certificate of proof, or a digital thumbprint, or part of the injection. This is stirring up those corny Conspirator Theorists that give people like, myself, a bad rep – thanks you whacky idiots!

They give all conspirator theorists a bad rap, because they jump to conclusions, take things out of context, and don't speak, before thinking a theory thru…logically & rationally!

Some of my various theories have been seen/heard as far-fetched, and they become truth, not long after! Which, makes it *Conspiracy Fact*, so ha, to the theories that have become fact!

Chapter 4

Today, April 28th, 2020, marks a historical event – even though the news is two years old…

The Pentagon released its first, official inferred, night vision video of a UFO – flying saucer. It's never been released before, officially. Nevertheless, I find the timing to be ironic, seeming how in this month (April of 2020), Utica & Rome, New York (upstate), has had footage of Orange Orbs flying in the skies – which has not been rejected by our government. Which, also is a historical announcement, all on its

own.

It makes you scratch your head,

and ask, *Why now?* I suppose the why,

and the when, doesn't matter. What

matter's is that they officially came

forward, and people can shut the "F"

up, about how flying saucers & Alien

orbs don't exist, when it is officially

stated, that they do!

I for one, cannot wait to get my

next camera, before the darn thing sells

out. If only my stimulus money, and

unemployment money rushes to be

cleared in my bank, so I can spend

nearly $900 on the darn thing! Then, I can finally rebuild, and update my Youtube channel!

The Power of Stupid (which is also the title of my next fictional book), is what this Virus should be renamed. Because, it is those who aren't infected with the virus, that have shown much stupidity! Perhaps, it's due to the lack of brain power, and activity from not working. Nevertheless, it's now a proven fact, humans are stupid…And it surprises me that we've made it as far as we have, as a race!

In Closing

Okay, okay. I know, this is the shortest book of the 3-part series. I am aware of this. Honestly, I wasn't intending on creating a third volume, but I thought, since I was making the third to put the first two volumes in a single copy, I should add new content – it only makes sense. However, I will not be publishing it as an individual book – it seems unnecessary.

Please check my books availability on

https://www.amazon.com/s?k=BOBBY+SIMONDS&ref=nb_sb_noss

135

I am constantly creating a new book, lately. Seeming how I am out of work, I am taking full advantage – and am not taking a 3-week-lapse-period in between books. Granted this series is short, I did recently release Volume 5 of, ***Bobby's Creative Photography***. Therefore, if my count is correct, this book makes 6 since I've been out since March!

This book makes 77 on my list, and I've only been self-publishing since April of 2014! It's been a long time. Perhaps, since this month is my anniversary of my first book being published, it could explain why the excessive creations!

I will hopefully get my website back online. I have an annual lease on my domain name, https://bobbysimonds.com/ Therefore, you don't have to worry about it being used by a wanna-be, of myself! Thanks for reading, I couldn't move forward without your support!

Please be courteous, and leave a two-second review – good or bad. Shoot me a private message on instant messenger on Facebook. I'm usually checking once a day!

Stay safe, and watch for the

signs that could be dooming your

bubble.

www.ingramcontent.com/pod-product-compliance
Lightning Source LLC
Chambersburg PA
CBHW051459250726
48655CB00001B/490